Bariatric Diet

Dietary Advice Before, and After Gastric Sleeve Weight Loss Surgery

By

Nicola Curtis

Understand and Disempower the Bully: You Are Good As You Are

ISBN: 9781521458839

Warning and Disclaimer

Publisher contact

Skinny Bottle Publishing

books@skinnybottle.com

SKINNY BOTTLE

Introduction

These days, there is so much focus on appearance and health that it is no wonder that we are more aware than ever before about our bodies. There are an upside and a downside to this, however – if you don't need to lose weight or change something about yourself, you could feel pressured into making changes that you don't need to make, and this can affect your self-esteem and overall health and wellbeing. On the other hand, if you are overweight and need to make changes, this awareness can be the one thing which pushes you towards the right avenue for you.

The fact you have picked up this book basically tells us that you are either seriously considering bariatric surgery or have had it and you're seeking extra clarification on the diet you need to follow now that you have a new lifestyle to keep up; we say 'lifestyle', because once you have had surgery of this kind, either a gastric band or a sleeve or even a gastric bypass, you're on this new regime for life. You need to know what to eat, and you need to know how to eat it. You even need to know how to prepare it and cook it.

Health isn't rocket science, but you need to re-educate yourself in terms of what healthy choices are and what unhealthy choices are in order to create habits that help you follow this diet to the letter.

Of course, following your new bariatric diet for life shouldn't be difficult if you are in the right mindset to begin with, e.g. you have made the decision to have this invasive surgical procedure for you and your heath alone, and therefore you are determined to do right by yourself and your body, and stay on the path to health and overall wellbeing.

Throughout this book, we are going to explore both sides of the coin: both what bariatric surgery is, how it works, what it is, and who is suitable for it, as well as what you should be doing after the surgery, i.e. the diet you need to follow. The primary aim is to give you a thorough overview of what you are about to embark upon, or help you come to terms with and process what you have already had done and help you stick to the right roads towards the rest of your healthy life.

First things first, let's explore briefly what bariatric surgery is.

Bariatric surgery is also known as weight loss surgery, but it is certainly not a quick fix for just anyone to have. It is a serious operation that needs careful planning and consideration, and it is only open to those who are severely overweight, obese, and who have tried everything else and failed.

A friend of mine recently underwent bariatric surgery, and truth be told, it has saved her life. She was seriously overweight. In fact, she was a walking advertisement for someone who could have keeled over right there and then – I'm not crossing lines by telling you this, she would tell you this herself. The great thing about it all, and the most admirable personality trait she has shown to date, is that she took the action she needed to take to save her life and stick around much, much longer for her kids.

Her weight loss surgery route wasn't easy, she had a gastric band operation, and she had a few complications afterward, but by following advice and sticking to her post-op diet to the letter, she is slim, and so much healthier than she has ever been.

If my friend isn't a walking advertisement for bariatric surgery and its fantastic effects for those who need it, I don't know who is!

The thing I didn't realize after her surgery is just how much her life had to change forever. I think many people are under the false assumption that once you have had the surgery, that's it, the weight is going to go quite quickly, and you're free to enjoy all the wonderful foods and beverages in the world from there on with no downsides.

Wrong!

The decision to have bariatric surgery is a decision to change your life completely and make lifestyle changes which will be far-reaching for the rest of your days. If you go back to your unhealthy eating habits, you are going to make yourself ill, totally undo all the good your surgery carried out, and probably waste an awful lot of money in the process.

You need to make a commitment to health, you need to review your relationship with food, you need to learn about nutrition, and you need to make friends with exercise. Forever.

So, wherever you are in your bariatric surgery story, whether you're at the start, or you're just post-op, this book is going to hold your hand through the whole process, leading you out the other side of the tunnel towards a much brighter and healthier future. We're going to give you a reiteration of bariatric surgery and what it is, we're going to explain the stages after the procedure so you know what you can and can't eat and so you know how you can eat it, and we're also going to give you some ideas to create your own ideas to enjoy whilst you're healing.

The bariatric diet isn't that restrictive once you know what you can and can't have and once you know how to twist it to make it not only delicious but super-healthy too.

All About Bariatric Surgery

We've talked about the fact that bariatric surgery is not a decision to take lightly, but for those who are suitable, this is a form of surgery which is life-changing in so many ways. Of course, like anything in life, there are various different types and options available, and it's important to understand them properly, not only to identify which is the best for you but also to know more about the surgery you have had or are considering having.

First things first, let's explore what bariatric surgery is in its most basic forms before we can move onto what this book is primarily about – the diet you need to follow after the surgery. Nobody should go into this half-heartedly, so let's give you the information you need, first of all, to help give you a totally clear, thorough overview of the journey you're about to take.

Bariatric surgery is the medical term for weight loss surgery, an operation which affects the way you take your food, which can then help you lose weight. Provided you follow the right guidelines, it can help you keep it off, too. Bariatric surgery is only for people who are dangerously obese, i.e. those who are so overweight that their health and life is in danger, and for those who have tried other ways to lose weight, but whose efforts have failed.

A doctor will have to speak with you and identify whether bariatric surgery is indeed for you before any decision is made. From there, the types of surgery will be discussed to explore the right option for you. Everyone is different, and that means that one option isn't always the best for all.

As a general rule, dangerously obese is often classifed as those who have a BMI (body mass index) of over 40. Before any doctor will agree to perform bariatric surgery, you will have to try and lose the weight yourself. If that doesn't work, or if it's simply too big a mountain to climb, you could be a candidate for a particular type of bariatric surgery.

Types of Bariatric Surgery

The main types of weight loss surgery (bariatric surgery) are:

- Gastric banding procedures

- Gastric bypass procedures

- Sleeve gastrectomy procedures

Whilst the end result is the same (weight loss), these are all subtly different in their own right, and that means they are all suitable for different people too.

Let's explore them in more detail.

Gastric Banding Procedure

A gastric banding procedure is done by reducing the size of the patient's stomach, and that means that less food is required in order to make the patient full. Obviously, that means that weight will be lost.

Gastric Bypass Procedure

In a gastric bypass procedure, the clue is in the name. The entire digestive system is given a re-route, bypassing most of the stomach. The patient, therefore, digests less food, and less food is also needed to create that feeling of being full. Again, weight is lost.

Sleeve Gastrectomy Procedure

This is probably the most drastic of all the bariatric procedures, and it is, therefore, the least used. Having said that, it is still often done, and it has a definite place in the world of bariatric procedures. For this book, we are going to concentrate on the first two more than anything else, but for information:

In a sleeve gastrectomy, a section of the stomach is actually removed, and therefore because the stomach is smaller, the patient needs less food to feel full. Again, the results are predictable.

As we mentioned previously, it is important to have a full and in-depth consultation to identify which form of bariatric surgery is the most suitable for you, if indeed this line of action is right for you at all. It often takes more than one consultation to come to a firm decision, because this is such a huge decision for a patient to make. From there, usually tests are done to ascertain suitability again, as well as counseling in terms of what to expect after the procedure.

From this, you can recognize the huge impact of this type of surgery overall.

The Potential Side Effects of Bariatric Surgery

As with any type of surgery, large or small, there are risks, and this also means that you need to be clear and informed of these before any decisions are made. Whenever you go under the surgeon's knife and are administered an anesthetic, you are putting yourself at risk, but the risk is small and manageable.

In terms of bariatric surgery, the main side effect risks include:

•   The risk of internal bleeding

•   Possible development of a DVT (deep vein thrombosis), ablood clot in the leg

•   The possibility of a blood clot or blockage in the lungs, also known as a pulmonary embolism

•   Death, but do bear in mind however that this is listed in the side effects, but it is highly unlikely

These side effects may sound grim, but it's important to weigh the likelihood versus the reality. These things can happen, but provided you have had a full consultation, you have a highly trained and professional surgeon, and you follow all advice given to you for both before and after the procedure, the risk of developing any of these side effects is very low indeed. Of course, we have mentioned that everyone is different, and that also means that the degree of side effect risk is different for everyone too. If you have any serious risk factors, e.g. family history of DVT, or you have suffered any medical conditions in the past, these should be disclosed to your surgeon at the very first consultation.

The Expected Results of Weight Loss Surgery

Yet again, we have to emphasize the same point – everyone is different! On a general note, however, weight loss surgery does have expected results, and your surgeon will be able to tell you what he or she expects for your particular circumstances.

Every single person who undergoes weight loss surgery needs to stick to the plan which was agreed to before the surgery, i.e. the lifestyle changes which are required after the procedure and are literally required FOR LIFE.

On average, the expected results for bariatric surgery include:

•   Gastric banding surgery patients are expected to lose around half of the amount of excess body weight they have

•   Gastric bypass surgery patients are expected to lose around two-thirds of the amount of excess body weight they have

Things to Consider

Before you decide to undergo bariatric surgery, ask yourself these questions:

•   Are you ready to change your lifestyle completely and stick to it for the rest of your life?

•   Are you dedicated to overall health?

•   Are you happy to incorporate regular exercise into your life?

•   Do you see weight loss surgery as a quick fix?

•   Do you understand the drastic nature of the procedure and its implications?

The diet you have to follow immediately after surgery can be tough for most patients because it is so restrictive, and you really have to educate yourself on what you can and can't have as well as how you can take your food. The diet then progresses to different stages, but when you reach the final stage, i.e. you have given your body the time it needs to heal and adjust, then you will be on the regime for the rest of your life. Even the slightest deviation could cause unpleasant side effects, and any prolonged changes could mean you put the weight back on, leaving the procedure totally useless and a waste of time.

On top of this, you need to realize that weight loss surgery could cause problems in your relationship. This might sound ridiculous because you're going to lose weight and become healthier, but many people experience excess skin which they weren't expecting, and this can in some cases lead to another procedure to get rid of this. You should also make sure that you are mentally prepared in the right way because some people who experience depression or anxiety can develop unrealistic expectations of what the procedure is going to do for them. When the results aren't what they wanted, they can become very down about the outcome.

Weight loss surgery is not a magic cure, but it is a way to change your life when other methods and options have failed.

Now that we know all about bariatric surgery, what it is, who is suitable for it, and the different types, we can now go on to talk about life after the surgery. The coming chapters are about the various stages of diet after the procedure, and it's important to state here and now that it is imperative to be strict in each one of them. Failure to do so can result in unpleasant effects and problems with your overall health.

Your Pre-Bariatric Surgery Diet

Before you have your surgery, you need to prepare your body and your stomach for what is about to happen. No matter what type of surgery you're going for, you basically need to empty your stomach, but be sure to keep your nutrient levels up in the days beforehand.

Prior to a gastric bypass surgical procedure, this is perhaps even more important. You will be asked to go onto what is known as a pre-op liquid diet. This is to reduce the amount of fat which is sitting around the spleen and the liver. This type of liquid diet must be strictly adhered to in the two weeks before your planned procedure. If you don't follow this diet, your operation could be canceled. It's that simple.

The liquid diet is not literal liquids as such, but it is very close to it. In the two weeks prior, you should eat only the following:

• Meal replacement shakes or protein shakes, which will probably be prescribed to you by your doctor. These are designed to give you the protein and the vitamins that your body needs whilst you are literally emptying your stomach of the undesirable things as well as the fat around your spleen and liver. If you don't take these as prescribed, you may become unwell, so make this a number one priority.

- Drinks which are totally sugar-free

- No drinks that contain caffeine – apologies but your coffee habit needs to be kicked

- No drinks which are carbonated, e.g. cola or anything fizzy

- Broth, but make sure it has no types of solid contained within it

- Vegetable juices

- Cream or rice or cream of wheat

On top of this, you need to know how to take these liquids: you should take them slowly and you should sip them.

It's quite likely that you will be given a plan to follow in this pre-operative time, and that means you are regularly getting the nutrition that your body needs. For instance, a sample could look something like this:

7 am – Meal replacement shake

8 am – Skimmed milk

9 am – Water

10 am – Another meal replacement shake

11 am – Water

12 pm – Broth

With a similar pattern for the rest of the day.

If you've read anything about diabetes management or any low carbohydrate diets on the market these days, such as Paleo, Atkins, or Keto, then you might know something about ketosis. The aim for this pre-bariatric surgery diet is to push your body into a ketosis state and to burn fat for energy rather than carbohydrates, which is the natural state. This means that your body shrinks down the excessive amount of fat it has stored up much faster, including the fat around the liver. The problem here however is that you need to ensure you're getting a good amount of protein, and this is why you should always take the meal replacement shakes in the way that you are prescribed them, because they contain a finely balanced amount of protein designed to give your body what it needs and no more than that.

Sticking to your pre-operative bariatric diet, whether for a gastric banding, sleeve, or a bypass, is the number one important thing you should have in your mind. Ensuring you are strict here gives your surgeon a better starting point, and that means you are much more likely to have a faster and smoother recovery.

The benefits of the pre-op bariatric diet are:

• The fat around the liver disappears fast

• Your body goes into ketosis, which means you will lose excessive abdominal fat way quicker, and this cuts down on what you need to work on during and after surgery

• Studies have shown that recovery time after the procedure is quicker and smoother when a pre-bariatric surgery diet has been adhered to properly

• There is no chance of your surgery being delayed due to improper diet beforehand

• You give yourself a head-start on the lifestyle and dietary changes you need to make after your procedure, putting yourself in the right headspace ahead of time

So, when you're struggling in the days leading up to your procedure because of the strict diet you are having to follow, remember the above benefit points and repeat them daily – stick them on your fridge if you need to!

There are slight differences between those who are undergoing the more drastic form of surgery, i.e. a gastric bypass, and those who are going the lesser form, e.g. banding, in terms of pre-operative diets, but the general ethos is the same. You should always stick to what your surgeon or doctor has prescribed for you, and you should do it to the letter. You are making a commitment to health and wellbeing for your future by having the surgery, and that means making a commitment to sticking to the rules before you even get to the operating table.

Now, you've done the pre-operative diet, the day of your surgery has passed, you've woken up from the anesthetic, and you need to follow the post-operative bariatric diet.

Are you in for a shock? Yes, to a degree, because it's going to be hard, so make peace with the fact now. If you followed your pre-operative diet, however, you will be in the right mindset, and you'll know pretty much what to expect and how it feels. The good news is that after your surgery you're not going to feel anywhere near as hungry as you did before it when you were following your pre-operative routine.

There is always a silver lining!

So, let's now go into what happens after your surgery.

Phase One - Life Immediately After Bariatric Surgery

Immediately after your bariatric surgery procedure, you are probably going to be feeling a little tender. The key here is to take everything slowly and steady. At this stage, you are allowing your body to heal, and you need to ensure that you don't stretch your stomach from eating the wrong kinds of food.

Eating small amounts of food which can be easily digested will help to re-train your stomach and slowly get used to the new circumstances. Your body will also learn to avoid the possible side effects which can come around after bariatric surgery, although much of this avoidance is going to be down to following the strict regime below.

This part of the journey is the most important because this is where irreparable damage can be done if the wrong route is followed. In terms of the different types of bariatric surgery and what you can and can't do, the journeys are slightly different, but not dissimilar.

If you fail to follow the post-operative bariatric diet properly, the following can occur:

- You will slow down or even stop the healing process altogether

- You will increase the risk of an infection at the operative site

- You will experience pain

- You may experience a very upset stomach, leading to diarrhea and vomiting

- If you have had a gastric band, you risk dislocating the band and having to go back for more surgery

- If you have had a gastric bypass, you could cause damage to the staple which is inside your body, and again, you may have to have more surgery, which could be more severe

Warning over, let's talk about the post-operative diet you need to follow and explore it all in more detail.

The First Phase After a Gastric Banding Procedure

The first phase after a gastric banding procedure lasts for the first four weeks after the procedure is carried out. In this phase you should not eat anything solid at all because by doing so, you will be putting extra pressure onto the band and you will damage it. Any damage at this point is going to be very difficult to fix, if it is fixable at all.

Liquids only for two weeks

For the first two weeks after your diet, you will be encouraged to consume only liquids that you can see through, e.g. clear liquids. Examples are water, tea, non-acidic fruit juice, broth, protein fruit beverages, sugar-free gelatins, etc. From there, you will be able to move onto a diet which includes more fluids that are not see through, including milk, protein shakes, and low fat cream soups.

Eat pureed food only as the next stage

This type of food is literally like the food you would give to a baby, but you can make it out of your favorite items and mix it with something wet, to create the puree. To puree the food, simply use a potato masher or a handheld blender if you want to make the process quicker and easier. A few examples of pureed food include:

- Ground lean meats (pureed using a blender)

- Beans

- Fish

- Eggs

- Soft fruit

- Cooked vegetables

- Cottage cheese

- Mashed potato

You can mix these up with anything wet, such water, skimmed milk, broth, or sugar-free juice

You should eat around 4 to 5 times per day, but you need to control the portion size, as anything too large could stretch your stomach, which is not what you need to be doing at any point after bariatric surgery. A portion is generally around the 100g mark or 4-6 tablespoons.

Remember to eat slowly. You need to chew as many times as you can before you swallow to ensure that the food is ground right down, even when pureed before it enters your mouth. Whenever you feel full, stop eating immediately. You might notice that fullness feels different after bariatric surgery, i.e. it might feel like a tightness or a fullness in your chest, rather than your stomach. That is because the band is located a little higher up than you are used to feeling.

Drink water

You should ideally drink 1.5 liters of water every day, however, do not drink whilst you are eating, and consume only in small glasses, around 100-200ml.

The main points to remember from this phase are:

- Only eat pureed food

- Drink water regularly in small amounts

- Do not drink water with meals

• Eat 4-5 times per day, in a portion of 100g or 4-6 tablespoons only

• Stop eating when you feel full – you may feel this as a tightness or fullness in your chest

• If you vomit a lot after you have finished eating, seek help. This could be because you are consuming too much food, or it may be that your band needs to be adjusted slightly.

The First Phase After a Gastric Bypass Procedure

The first phase after a gastric bypass procedure has a few differences to that found in a gastric banding procedure. For the first week, you can only consume liquids, no pureed foods or anything similar. The first phase within this procedure lasts for less than a gastric banding, around 2 weeks maximum. During that time you can have foods such as creamed soups, provided there are no lumps in them, e.g. cream of chicken, etc. These can be strained out to leave behind a creamy liquid to enjoy and put to bed any hunger pangs.

Only drink liquids for the first week

Whereas with a gastric banding, you can eat pureed food basically from the get-go, with a gastric bypass, this isn't the case. The first few days after the surgery, you can have:

• Broth

• Unsweetened juices

- Decaffeinated tea

- Decaffeinated coffee

- Skimmed milk

- Strained cream types of soup

- Sugar-free gelatin

- Sugar-free popsicles

Take your time

Make sure you take small sips, rather than big drinks, and take your time -- don't drink sip after sip. Once you feel that sense of fullness or tightness, again, you should stop. This tightness or fullness will be felt in the stomach area, rather than the chest, with a gastric bypass, because there is no band which sits slightly higher up. Learning to recognize fullness is key in this particular type of surgery.

Phase one of either type of procedure, as we mentioned, is the hardest of them all, but once you are past the first two to four weeks (four with a gastric band), then you can slowly start to incorporate different types of food and different frequencies. As with any surgery type, the first few weeks afterward is all about allowing your body to adjust and learn the new way to act and be. If you rush anything here, you are going to have complications. The main one that most people experience when they try to go too fast is vomiting. If this occurs repeatedly, it's important to seek medical help, whether this is due to a banding operation or a bypass.

Now, let's check out phase two.

Phase Two - Life After Bariatric Surgery

After the first phase, you can gradually begin to incorporate other types of food and liquid into your diet, slowly but surely. In terms of a gastric banding, this can happen after the fourth week and goes into the sixth week. For a gastric bypass, it is earlier, beginning after the second week until the fourth week.

As with the first phase, it's important to take things slowly and don't overeat or push your stomach to accept what it doesn't want to. The rule of stopping eating and drinking when you feel any fullness still applies and will continue to apply for the rest of your life. Recognizing genuine hunger is one of the key factors of avoiding weight gain in any diet. A lot of the time when you feel hungry, you're actually just thirsty, so this is something you should try to keep in mind.

In terms of what you can eat and how you should eat it during the second phase, however, let's check them out one by one.

The Second Phase After a Gastric Banding Procedure

Beginning at the fourth week, you can begin to change your diet a little. This is going to be similar to the first phase, but you can bring in foods which aren't pureed, but they should be soft. For instance, in the second phase you can try the following:

- Whole-wheat breakfast cereals mixed with skimmed milk

- Porridge with plenty of skimmed milk or water

- Mashed potato, with or without a little melted cheese for taste

- Soups, provided there are no hard lumps in it, e.g. hard potato, etc.

- Yoghurts

- Rice pudding

These give you an idea of the types of food you can enjoy during this phase and it does bring more variety into proceedings. In terms of liquids, things are much freer at this point, however everything you consume must be healthy, e.g. water should still be in small amounts, and milk should be skimmed, etc. Avoid anything with high sugar content, such as sweetened juices.

As before, these rules still apply:

- Chew your food until thoroughly mashed up before you swallow

- Eat 4-6 times per day, in small amounts

• Whenever you feel a sense of fullness or pressure in the chest, you are full and you should stop eating

• Do not drink whilst you are eating, as this will affect how you digest the food

• Drink plenty of water in small amounts throughout the day

• If you find that you are vomiting after meals, cut back a little on what you are eating or how often, and this should rectify the problem. However, again, this is also something you should check out with your doctor if it is persistent. Because a band is something which can be adjusted, it is often a case of trial and error in the beginning.

The Second Phase After a Gastric Bypass Procedure

The second phase after a gastric bypass procedure comes a little sooner than it does in the case of a gastric banding, and you can begin introducing pureed food around the two-week mark. Because in the case of a gastric bypass you can only drink liquids in the first two weeks, you are not now incorporating soft foods, but pureed foods. As we mentioned in the first phase of a gastric banding procedure, a few pureed foods you can try include:

• Ground lean meats (pureed using a blender)

• Beans

• Fish

• Eggs

- Soft fruit

- Cooked vegetables

- Cottage cheese

- Mashed potato

Make sure you mix with liquids when you are pureeing, as this will make the whole process more effective and easier, and you can try skimmed milk, water, broth, etc. Quantities to consume are the same as the first phase of the banding procedure, i.e. 100g portions, 4-5 times a day.

This particular phase of a gastric bypass procedure is basically the first phase of a banding, and the healing process is a little slower in the case of this procedure. The reason for this is because you have rerouted your digestive system, rather than simply shrinking it with the aid of a band, and that involves the healing of scar tissue and other internal problems. Taking it steady is therefore imperative, and this will stop the chances of any damage or side effects from occurring.

We are going to talk about exercise after bariatric surgery in more detail in a later chapter, but towards the end of the second phase is a good time to commence light exercise routines. Always check this out with your doctor before going ahead with anything particularly strenuous, as you don't want to cause any problems with the internal healing, but overall, starting to move around and get your blood and heart pumping is a great idea and is something which will certainly help you in your weight loss endeavours.

It's also important to remember that whilst the whole point of weight loss surgery is pointed out within the name (weight loss), the first two phases are about healing, not weight loss. You will find that you do lose weight very quickly in these phases, but that is not the key aim. First, you are healing, and then you are losing weight towards a manageable and healthier BMI for your body. Rushing and following a crash diet at this point, even with the restrictive nature of the post-bariatric surgery, could cause damage and also make you rather unhealthy and unwell too.

Phase Three - Life After Bariatric Surgery

Phase three is basically the phase that you remain in for the rest of your life, and it is at this point where you will develop healthy eating habits that will see you towards a healthy and sustainable weight. You will find that the amount of weight you lose during the few weeks after this will be dramatic, and that should certainly do a lot for your confidence overall.

The diet at this point is the same for both gastric band and gastric bypass procedures. You should remain eating small meals and then stop eating when you feel a sense of being full. If you overeat, you are not going to lose weight, and you will probably end up vomiting rather unpleasantly. Your body is going to revolt rather spectacularly at this point if you push yourself, so stick within your limits, and the results will be very pleasing indeed.

The third phase begins at six weeks, and as we mentioned, goes on for the rest of your life. This is the point where you make sustainable lifestyle changes, and you are now ready to adopt a diet which is long-term and easy to stick to, whilst also being enjoyable too. By this point, if you have had a gastric band, then it is probably adjusted and is right for your body, and you should also have noticed that you need much less food than before to satisfy your appetite.

At this point you need to remember the following points:

• Learn about nutrition and what is good for your body. Reading food labels is a good way to go, but sticking with fresh and healthy produce is ideal.

• Three meals per day is enough.

• Snacking should not be needed because you shouldn't be feeling hungry.

• By the third phase you can eat solid foods, and these will make you feel fuller quicker than in the first two stages.

• Eat slowly – cut your food into small pieces and chew them thoroughly and slowly before swallowing.

• Stop eating when you are full. In the case of a gastric banding, again, you may feel this in your chest, as a tightening or a fullness, but wherever you feel it, stop when you do feel it!

• Overeating will cause you to be in pain and it may cause you to vomit.

• Avoid drinking with your meals, even water – this is because the liquid is flushing out your stomach as you are eating, so you're actually consuming more calories. It's best to avoid any liquids for half an hour before you eat, and for one hour afterward. After that make sure you drink plenty of water to stay hydrated.

• Watch what you are eating – full fat, high-calorie content drinks should be out, and that includes cola, alcohol, fruit juices which are sweetened, and milkshakes. Stick to zero calorie beverages, skimmed milk, and water.

• High sugar foods need to be avoided, and this includes cakes and biscuits. The reason for this is because sugary foods affect your digestive system and causes you to release extra insulin. This then causes symptoms of Dumping Syndrome, including nausea, diarrhea, light-headedness, and vomiting.

The Importance of Vitamins & Minerals

Most bariatric surgery patients take vitamin and mineral supplements because this ensures that the right amount of vitamins and minerals are taken in and that there is no deficiency occurring anywhere in the body. This is obviously a personal decision, but most patients do take a mixture of:

• Multi-vitamin supplements

• Calcium supplements

• Iron supplements

The dosage depends on the person, i.e. whether male or female, weight, height, etc., so this is something you should be checking with your doctor to ensure you are taking the right amount, not too much or too little. Obviously, getting plenty of fresh fruit and fresh vegetables will also help, as well as skimmed milk in your diet.

Overall, a healthy and balanced diet includes a mixture of the five main food groups. These include:

• Protein – You can get enough protein from lean chicken, fresh fish products, free range eggs, and beans. These are filling and healthy options to enjoy and can also be enjoyed with many other delicious foods.

• Dairy products – You need to be careful how much dairy you are consuming and keep everything low fat, i.e. skimmed milk and cheese and yogurt which is low in fat.

• Carbohydrates – You might have carbs down as the devil, but they do need to be in your diet to a degree. Carbs are found in foods such as bread, cereals, and potatoes. In order to get the most nutrition from these foods, as well as sticking to overall health, go for whole grain varieties.

• Fresh fruit and vegetables – The fresher the better, the brighter the better. This should be your mantra. Around five portions of fruit and veg per day should be your aim.

• Fats – You do need to keep fat to a minimum, but it's important to have some in your diet also. When you are cooking, if you use a small amount of oil (olive, of course), then you are basically getting the fat intake that you need for that day without having to think about anything else.

Mixing up your diet to include these groups whilst also cooking them in the right way will give you everything you need from your food and drink. Remember our section about the possibility of including a vitamin and mineral supplement into your diet, as this will boost your intake, and make sure that you are getting everything you really need, without missing out.

Learning About Healthy Food Choices

Because you are on this diet for the rest of your life, it's important to develop healthy habits which help you gain variety and enjoyment from what you eat. Food is such a socially important part of our lives, as well as the way we gain fuel for our bodies to work effectively, so it's vital to make sure that we mix up what we eat, whilst also ensuring that whatever we do consume is healthy.

It's really not rocket science, but these rules will help you realize what is healthy and what isn't:

- Stick to lean meat

- Cook on the grill, rather than frying

- Olive oil is always better

- Saturated fat is a big no-no

- Five portions of fruit and vegetables per day is recommended

- Avoid anything high in sugar, e.g. hidden sugars in fruit juices, etc

- Skimmed milk and low-fat yogurts will help you get your daily calcium intake

- Decaffeinated tea and coffee is the way forward

- Celery is a good option when you are craving something salty and keeps you from reaching for those potato chips

• One square of dark chocolate should be enough to starve off any sweet cravings

• When you feel hungry, try drinking water and see if the feeling disappears – this will tell you whether you are truly hungry or not

• Exercise can also take away hunger pangs that are not real

• Check out food labels, as these will help you understand the real content of packaged foods. Eating home cooked foods is always more nutritional than ready meals you buy from the supermarket

Eating healthy is not really difficult. It's about avoiding fatty foods and going for foods which are fresh and brightly colored – it's that simple!

How to Cook Your Food in a Healthy Way

Cooking your food is really half the battle. Even the healthiest of vegetables can be made unhealthy if you cook it in the wrong way! We know that eating small meals is key, but if you fry them, you're adding saturated fat into the equation, and this is in no way healthy. The key? Grilling!

Now, if you do fry, you need to be careful what you fry it in. Olive oil is always better, but you need to stick to a small amount for this to be healthy. Sunflower oil is bad, general cooking oil is bad, olive oil is good – remember that mantra. There is a reason that the Mediterranean Diet is considered ultra-healthy.

Cutting foods into small, easily digestible pieces is also key because this not only helps the food cook much easier and quicker, but it is also easier for you to chew and digest. When you are cooking, also avoid adding extra salt, as most foods have enough salt content within them to be enough for your daily allowance.

So, to sum it up into easy to remember points:

• Grill everything, rather than fry

• If you must fry, shallow fry only and use olive oil

• Cut food into smaller pieces, to make cooking easier and better whilst also retaining vitamins and minerals,

• Do not add extra salt

• Chili is a good addition, because not only does it add flavor, but it also helps to burn calories

• When sourcing fresh fruit and veg, the brighter, firmer, and fresher, the better

Bariatric Diet Meal / Snack Ideas

It's all very well and good telling you what you can and can't eat, how to cook it, and how to chew it, but it's not so easy to come up with ideas of what you can consume on a daily basis. You have had surgery, and yes you need to be careful, but you should also mix and match your diet to give you some variation as well as make sure that your body gets the variation and mixture of vitamins and minerals it still very much needs from the food and drinks you consume.

We're now going to give you a few recipe ideas and plans on what to eat at the different stages of the bariatric diet, to give you some inspiration, and to help you see that you can still enjoy foods, despite the restrictions placed upon you during the healing process.

Remember to adapt these suggestions to the stage you're on, so you don't push your healing too far. In terms of the pureed food stage of the diet, many of these suggestions will serve you very well and give you plentiful enjoyment from your diet, without being bored or unsatisfied.

Remember, this is by no means and exhaustive list, but it will help you see that life doesn't have to be dull and restrictive whilst you're healing and changing your entire outlook on food and beverages.

Idea 1 - Frozen Frappuccino

If you're a total coffee nut and you're missing your daily hit, especially of the cold, rather calorie-ridden variety from High Street coffee stores, you can save cash and keep up with your diet by making your own!

Ingredients

- 3 tbsp brewed coffee

- 3 tbsp Low fat, low sugar milk (e.g. almond milk)

- 6 tbsp thick, 0% fat yogurt

- 150ml Sweetener

- 1 tbsp cocoa powder

- 1 cup Ice

Method

- Into a blender, place the coffee, yogurt, milk, and sweetener, as well as the ice and cocoa, and combine until totally smooth

- Pour into a glass and enjoy!

Idea 2 - A Smoothie to Give You 5 a Day

We all know that we should be eating a range of fruits and vegetables every single day, whether we are on a bariatric diet or not, but it can be hard to fit them in! This smoothie takes away the stress, giving you your five a day with ease. It is also a delicious and totally bariatric diet-friendly option.

Ingredients

1 apple

1 pear

10g spinach leaves

5 tbsp coconut milk, low fat

A quarter of a peeled avocado, chopped up

150ml fresh orange juice

Method

• Make sure the apple is de-cored and cut into small pieces

• Take your blender and combine all ingredients together until totally combined and smooth

• Pour into a glass and enjoy!

Idea 3 – Spicy Soup

A soup is an ideal meal for a cold day, but even if it's not the middle of winter, soup is a great way to fill up, warm up, and basically get the nutrition you need in one hit.

Ingredients

- 1 onion, chopped

- 2 leeks, sliced

- 450g swede, chopped

- 450g carrots, chopped

- Salt

- Pepper

- 2 garlic cloves, crushed

- 2tsp curry powder

- 1.2 liters of vegetable stock

- Lemon juice, just a squeeze

Method

- Spray a pan with low-fat cooking spray and allow to heat up

- Cook the onions, leeks, swede, carrots and season with salt and pepper

- Cook for around half an hour, until the contents of the pan, are soft

- Add the garlic and the curry powder, and continue to cook for another 2 minutes

- Add the stock and allow the contents to boil

- Turn the heat down and simmer for 15 minutes

- Remove the soup from the pan and place in a blender, combining until smooth

- Add back to the pan and add the lemon juice

- Warm up again for a couple of minutes and serve

Idea 4 – Frozen Yoghurt Strawberry Popsicles

If it's a hot day and you're wanting a cooldown, or perhaps you're having a sweet craving, these little frozen delights will tick the box.

Ingredients

- 500g fat-free yogurt

- 25 strawberries

Method

- Place the yogurt and the strawberries into a food process and combine until the contents are smooth

- Take your popsicle molds and pour in the mixture, attaching the bottom sticks

- Freeze for around 4-6 hours – the contents should be firm and frozen

- Remove the mold and enjoy!

Idea 5 – Cheesy Garlic Cauliflower

If you're a lover of cauliflower cheese, you'll probably be lamenting the loss of this from your diet, but never fear! You can incorporate it into the puree stage of your diet with ease, with just a few tweaks.

Ingredients

- Frozen cauliflower florets, 1 bag

- 1 tsp butter

- 1 tsp salt

- 0.25 tsp garlic powder

- 0.25 cup mozzarella cheese (shredded)

- 0.25 cup parmesan cheese

- 0.25 cup milk

Method

- Place all ingredients into a blender and combine until totally smooth

- Pour into an oven-proof dish

- Sprinkle extra mozzarella cheese over the top

- Place in the oven to bake for around half an hour, or microwave for 90 seconds

Idea 6 – Delicious Egg Salad

You will easily fulfill some of your protein needs with this pureed version of the famous egg salad, making it an ideal snack or lunch choice.

Ingredients

- 2 eggs

- 1 tsp mayonnaise

- 0.5 tsp brown mustard

- Salt

- Pepper

Method

- Place everything into a blender and combine until smooth

- Serve!

Idea 7 – Ricotta & Lemon

This ideal treat is ideal for when you're craving something sweet, but it also packs a protein punch, thanks to the ricotta cheese.

Ingredients

- Part skimmed ricotta cheese, 15oz tub

- One lemon's zest

- Half a lemon's juice

- 1.5 tsp vanilla extract

- 4 packs of Splenda or sweetener

Method

- Combine all ingredients in the blender

- Serve!

Idea 8 – Spiced Pumpkin Soup

We already have one soup on our suggestion list, but this one is a classic, and can easily be incorporated into your bariatric diet efforts, without cheating in the slightest!

Ingredients

- 1 onion, chopped

- 2 garlic cloves, chopped

- 5cm fresh ginger, grated

- 2 tsp curry powder

- 750g pumpkin, cut into small pieces

- 4000g low-fat coconut milk

- 400ml vegetable stock

- Salt

- Black pepper

Method

- Spray a pan with low-fat cooking spray and allow it to heat up

- Cook the onion, for around 4 minutes until softening

• Add in the garlic, ginger and the curry powder and continue to cook for around a further minute

• Now, add the pumpkin, the stock, and the coconut milk

• Bring the mixture to the boil

• Turn the heat down and allow to simmer for around 12 minutes – ensure the pumpkin is softened

• Pour the mixture into a blender and blitz to combine

• Season with salt and pepper

• Return to the pan and heat up before serving

Idea 9 – Buffalo Chicken

This is a seriously tasty meal which will certainly hit your taste-buds. If you can't find canned chicken where you live, regular chicken can be pureed provided it is cooked beforehand.

Ingredients

- 1 can of chicken

- 1 tbsp blue cheese crumbles/croutons

- 2 tbsp ranch salad dressing

- 1 tbsp buffalo sauce

- Salt

- Pepper

Method

- Combine all ingredients together in a blender

- Ensure the crumbles/croutons are totally combined

- Serve!

Idea 10 – Winter Squash Casserole

You don't have to forego the winter warming casserole just because you're in the middle of the puree stage of your bariatric recovery diet, and this squash casserole is simply delicious.

Ingredients

- 1 can of squash

- 2 tbsp cream cheese

- 0.5 tsp garlic powder

- Salt

- Pepper

- 1 tsp butter

- 1 tbsp cheddar cheese (shredded)

Method

- Puree all ingredients in your blender until totally combined

- Transfer the mixture into an oven-proof dish

- Sprinkle over a little more shredded cheddar cheese

- Place in the microwave for around 90 seconds, or in the oven for half an hour

- Serve!

Idea 11 – Avocado, Chicken & Potato

This mixture gives you some serious health benefits, thanks to the superfood addition of avocado, whilst also getting your protein hit from the chicken.

Ingredients

- 1 potato, peeled and cut into small pieces

- 2oz chicken breast, skinned and boned

- 0.5 avocado, stoned and peeled

- 2 tsp fat-free milk

- Salt

- Pepper

Method

- Boil or steam the potato until soft

- Steam the chicken – you can do this with the potato if you like

- Place the potato and chicken into a blender with the avocado, milk, and seasoning

- Blend together until completely smooth

- Enjoy!

Idea 12 – Delicious Chili

Everyone loves a chili, and just because you're on your bariatric diet doesn't mean you can't enjoy this most delicious of dishes!

Ingredients

- 1lb ground beef

- 1 can pinto beans

- Chili seasoning, the low sodium variety, 1 packet

Method

- Cook the beef until browned

- Add the chili seasoning and a little water and combine

- Add the pinto beans and mix together

- Simmer for around 10 minutes

- Place the mixture into the blender and combine until smooth

- Enjoy!

Idea 13 – Cheesy Lasagna

Again, a classic which is adapted to make it perfect for the puree stage of the post-bariatric surgery diet.

Ingredients

- 0.75 cup of ricotta cheese, fat-free variety

- 0.25 cup of spaghetti sauce

- 0.25 tsp oregano

- 0.25 tsp basil

- 2 egg whites

- 1/3 cup mozzarella cheese, the low-fat variety

Method

- Mix together the ricotta, the egg whites, oregano, and basil, and ensure all combined well

- Transfer the mixture into an oven-proof dish

- Pour the spaghetti sauce over the top

- Sprinkle with mozzarella cheese

- Bake for 20 minutes until the cheese is bubbling

Idea 14 – Refreshing Ice Tea

Diets aren't all about food, and this bariatric-friendly try on the classic ice tea refreshment will have your thirst sated.

Ingredients

- 1 lemon/ginger tea bag

- 250ml hot water

- 3 tbsp grapefruit juice

- Ice

- Lemon slices

Method

- Place the tea bag in the hot water

- Leave it alone for around 5 minutes

- Remove the tea bag and let the 'tea' go cold

- Add the grapefruit juice and stir to combine

- Place ice in a glass and pour the mixture into the glass

- Decorate the glass with lemon slices

Idea 15 – Tomato, Lentil and Mint Soup

Delicious with a capital D, whether you're following a bariatric diet or not! This dish ah Turkish origins and certainly has a tasty tang to it.

Ingredients

- 1 onion, chopped

- 1 garlic clove, chopped

- 400g chopped tomatoes (can)

- 400g lentils (can)

- A little fresh mint, chopped

- 600ml vegetable stock

- Salt

- Black pepper

Method

- Coat a frying pan with low-fat cooking spray

- Cook the onion and garlic for around 5 minutes, until soft

- Add the tomatoes, lentils, mint, salt, pepper, and the stock and combine

- Allow the mixture to boil

• Turn the heat down and cover, allowing to simmer for around 20 minutes

• Blend the mixture before serving

These 15 snack and meal ideas should have given you a good overview of just how you can adjust the stages of the bariatric diet to still be delicious and cut out the restriction to a degree. Most of these recipes are ideal for the puree stage, no matter what type of bariatric surgery you have had. Remember to look at the calorie intake you are having throughout the day in your other meals, but the great thing about these suggestions is that they are using fresh ingredients, many of which are high in nutrition, and that is basically what healthy eating is all about.

You will feel full quite quickly when you begin to start eating pureed dishes in particular, after the liquid-only stage of your diet. This is normal and is not something to be upset or distressed about. You should simply stop eating when you are full and remember not to overload your stomach; otherwise, you risk complications, and you will also experience rather unpleasant side effects too.

Take small mouthfuls, chew properly before swallowing, and above all else, enjoy what you eat! You've worked hard, and whilst you need to be mindful of what you're eating, there's no reason why you can't adapt a lot of your former favorite dishes into bariatric-friendly foods, provided you look at calorie counts and you puree it down, especially at this stage of the recovery.

The Internet is a fantastic place for inspiration, as well as forums where you will be able to get extra support from other bariatric surgery patients, many of whom will be all too happy to swap recipe ideas, as you all try and seek out some super-delicious creations to fit in with your diet.

Be careful of packaged meals and other types of foods which claim to be bariatric-diet friendly – it's always best to cook these things yourself rather than buying them in a tin, frozen package, or otherwise, because a) you don't really know what's in them unless you truly understand food labels, b) they're highly unlikely to be as healthy as they claim, and c) when fresh ingredients are frozen or left for too long, they can lose their nutrient value, and you will be left with a less than desirable meal, when you are probably very much looking forward to it!

It's all about experimentation, so allow yourself to get creative!

Conclusion

We have now covered everything we can about the post-bariatric diet, as well as giving you plentiful information on the subject itself and plentiful ideas for delicious meals to try yourself.

You might not have had your surgery yet, you might be thinking about it, or you might be sitting in the hospital recovering from your particular procedure. Whatever your point in this journey, what really matters is that you take it slowly and you do everything that is expected of you in order to help the healing process and help make this one of the best decisions you ever made.

A quick chat with my friend about her bariatric surgery confirmed what I always suspected from my research – bariatric surgery is not just about a quick fix, and it isn't about something which is even going to just take a few months and hey presto! You're skinny! It's about a lifestyle change that will never end, and it has to be something you're totally and utterly committed to, in order to get the right results and to do your body the justice it requires. Do not put your body through the stress and trauma of surgery of this kind, only to make it suffer by overeating or making poor food choices – you've come this far! We've talked about and shown you some delicious recipes, and that alone should show you that you aren't going to be waving goodbye to deliciousness!

So, if you haven't had your surgery yet, and you're thinking about embarking on this journey, the first thing you need to do is head to see your doctor and discuss your choices. Take their advice seriously and don't jump into this head first. Try a few other things first, e.g. diet and exercise, and willpower alone. If that doesn't work, yes, you may just be the right kind of person to successfully put this bariatric surgery journey to the test.

When you are discussing the type of surgery to have, e.g. gastric banding or a gastric bypass, as the two most popular types, be sure to weigh up the pros and cons of each.

Gastric Banding Pros & Cons

Pros:

• The band is adjustable so you can be sure that you will find the right result for you

• Less invasive than a gastric bypass

• Generally includes a shorter hospital stay

• Has the lowest rate of postoperative complications

• It is a reversible and adjustable procedure

• Has a high success rate

Cons:

• Serious surgery that should be thought about in detail before embarking on it

• Is associated with a slower weight loss than other procedures

• Some patients don't like the feeling of having something 'foreign' inside their body

• The feeling of fullness is felt in the chest, which can be strange

• There may be a period of time when the band needs to be adjusted once or twice

Gastric Bypass Pros & Cons

Pros

• Suppresses hunger in many ways, which makes the whole weight loss process easier

• Highly successful and commonly requested surgery

• There is no 'foreign' item with the body and hunger/fullness will be felt in the stomach, making it easier to recognize when enough food has been consumed

Cons

• An invasive procedure

• Can have a longer recovery time than a gastric banding procedure

• Longer hospital stay required

• A slightly higher chance of postoperative complications

• Irreversible procedure

Choosing the right procedure for your personal circumstances will mean that the road to your weight loss is easier and therefore is more successful overall. Listen to your healthcare professional and make sure that you discuss each in turn, asking any questions you may have.

All that is left to say at this point is good luck. Whether you have had your surgery, you're about to, or you're thinking about having it, bariatric surgery is something which will change your life for the better, provided you adhere to the diet and put your all into the after-care issues.

Life is quite simply too short to struggle, and if your health is on the line, there is only one answer to the whole conundrum. Be like my friend, the one who is now slim, happy, and healthy, and well on the way to achieving everything she ever wanted, with nothing holding her back.

Win a free

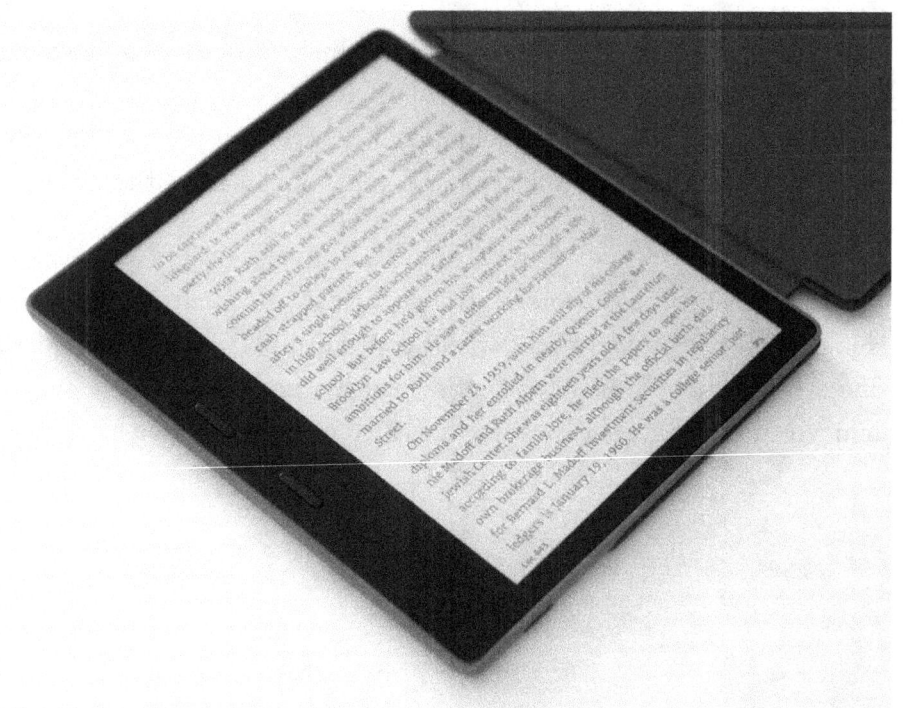

kindle
OASIS

Let us know what you thought of this book to enter the sweepstake at:

booksfor.review/bariatric

[Page intentionally left blank]

[Page intentionally left blank]